'Til Death
Do Us Part

A Story of a Lifetime of Devotion

by

Suzanne Johnson

ISBN-13: 978-1475077100
ISBN-10: 1475077106

www.AlzStory.com

Second Edition 2012

Dedication

To My Dad,
My Life-long Hero.

Oh the comfort,
the inexpressible comfort
of feeling safe with a person,
having neither to weigh thoughts
nor measure words, but pouring them
all right out, just as they are.
Certain that a fateful hand will
Take and sift them
keep what is worth keeping
And with kindness
Blow the rest away.

~ Dinah Maria Mulock Craik

Forward

This is an exceptional personal love story and the photos add a wonderful level of sentiment. Although Alzheimer's is a devastating condition, the writer demonstrates how Alzheimer's steals the mind but is unable to steal the heart. This story is a wonderful example of enduring strength, courage and love in the face of Alzheimer's. The Johnson family held on to her memories for her like a mother holds on to her child. This is a very intimate and very touching account of a heart-breaking disease.

Dr. Ethelle G. Lord, DM
President and Professional Alzheimer's Coach
http://remembering4you.com

Introduction

I have often been asked what made me decide to write my book. To be honest, it was never intended to be a publicized work. I began to write my thoughts a few days following my mother's death to ease my own personal grieving. Writing and journaling has always been an outlet for me so I used it to ease the pain. During the course of my mother's illness, my father took daily notes regarding her condition. Sometimes a line or two was all he would enter maybe saying she would not eat today, or this was a good day, but there were also words of hope, followed by discouragement and pain. After 15 years of caring for her, Dad had quite a compilation of notes. After Mom died, I asked him if I could look them over and it was through his writing along with thoughts of my own that I based a memoir that I presented to him and a few close family relations. I was then encouraged to take my story a step further with the hope of offering some understanding to others in similar situations. But this is the story of one care givers journey. Many others have had to make different choices and agonizing decisions to follow their heart and suit their needs. I can simply offer what I witnessed as a daughter.

Writing this book also gave me a chance to fight back in my own small way by speaking out and raising awareness of this gripping disease of sad goodbyes. The relentless symptoms only become worse with time, wearing down its victims and anyone else personally involved. The disease itself is shameless and shows no mercy to those afflicted. But it doesn't end there. It is cruelly passed on through a mutated gene to family members to reignite its thunderous course.

Therefore, I have decided to write this book to share my mother's experience and to honor my father's devotion towards her.

My parents met in 1941 while my mother was in nursing school. A classmate introduced her to my Dad on a blind date and the rest was history. Ironically enough, the first date they had was a trip to the same lake where she spent her last days.

They were married in 1945. My mother had become an RN. During the war, they were beginning to draft nurses, so the joke has always been that my mother 'had' to get married to dodge the draft. It was a small quiet ceremony; in fact my father went to work the next day. He was employed at the Enterprise Foundry in Lewiston that was founded by his father in the early 1900's. They married and had 3 daughters. Life had its hardships but they always seemed to find a way through the difficult times.

My mother was raised on a farm in Farmington and knew the value of a dollar. She had many talents and was successful at anything she set her mind to. Her skills included knitting elaborate sweaters, sewing beautiful clothes, upholstering, furniture refinishing as well as excelling in such sports like tennis, golf (hole in one at Fairlawn), skiing and I even remember the time she participated in an all-women's broom hockey game. All of these skills and memories were gradually swept away like dust by the shadow of Alzheimer's.

It was not until 1988 that my mother began showing signs of confusion and indecision. The 3 of us had grown up and had moved out of the house so I was not fully aware of how it started but my father remembers all too well. Mom had always been the book keeper of the family and suddenly she became unable to properly write out a check. Numbers did not make sense. Simple forgetfulness was blamed on getting older but it became more of a concern as events became more serious. One day my parents had gone grocery shopping. They unloaded and packed away several bags of groceries. It was only a few moments later when my mother asked where the groceries had gone.

She seemed to know there was something wrong at this early stage because she began writing things down and clipping out articles on memory loss. She once told me "not to get old because it's just not fun."

My father is from the old French Canadian generation. Very strong willed, methodical, proud and hard working. House cleaning, cooking and raising children were not a part of his agenda. Women's lib was unheard of at the time and my mother was just as happy in her place at home with the children anyway. It was a compromising union of give and take that worked well for them. When the diagnosis was made, changes took place that my father would never have thought possible had he the chance to peer into the future.

As she became unable to perform familiar tasks, he took on the responsibility of managing the household but still tried to engage her in the routines as much as possible. They made beds together, folded clothes, washed dishes etc. I suppose his motto was 'Hold on to as much as you can for as long as you can.' My mother had always kept a spotless house and even during her illness she still found the urge to scrub and polish. My father saw her scrubbing and wiping the kitchen sink one morning using repetitive motions. He told her she was a doing a "great job" and she replied, "I learned it from you!" In spite of this tremendous role reversal, he was determined to do everything in his power to offer my mother support, love, respect and devotion while preserving her dignity until the bitter end. This was so important to him. Mom always looked neat and clean wherever they went. It made his life look simple. No one witnessed the early morning baths, the physical transfers from bed to chair, the falls she took, the daily dressing and personal care that took place. When she became incontinent, the issues became even more complicated and taxing but he never complained.

One of the earlier doctor visits involved a local neurologist who encouraged Dad to get his affairs in order and start making arrangements for my mother. He blatantly spoke about the signs and symptoms of Alzheimer's in the presence of my mother, mentioning eventual nursing home care. Dad was very sensitive to this and it only managed to strengthen his resolve about keeping her at home. Although he understood that someday, something may happen to him and she would be forced to live in a nursing home, he was adamant about giving up on her if there was any way he could keep her at home with him. In the end, he was allowed this humble request. She died peacefully in the serenity of their summer cottage by the lake.

For the victim, there's also a stage of shame and covering up. My father in law also suffered from Alzheimer's and on the day he was to be evaluated, he asked to bring along his little book that he kept of himself with resumes of his accomplishments to show the doctor so he wouldn't think he was 'ignorant.' It must be so difficult when you know things are not right but can't understand why. Patience, understanding and compassion are so important at this stage and one of the best ways to express this is through touch.

Words don't always make sense and thoughts are soon forgotten but the message through touch is so meaningful and simple to give. When I stayed with my Mom to relieve my Dad, I would often massage her legs, her arms, her shoulders. There seemed to be so little else to offer and it did seem to have a calming effect. Sometimes the patient will develop tremors or perform repetitive motions. A soothing touch can relax these impulses and reaffirm that someone is there. But the best piece of advice I can offer care givers is to take care of yourselves and accept help when it is offered. Sometimes people don't know what to say and will ask, "Is there anything I can do?" Use this as a golden opportunity and make the suggestion yourself. Tell them you would like the chance to go to a movie, visit a friend or family member, go to the library or just out for a walk. My Dad always wanted to do it all and it's fortunate that he survived as well as he did. I wish he could have accepted more help because the care is exhausting. His determination must have carried him through although caring for a loved one at home is not always the best choice or even physically possible. Keeping Mom at home was Dad's personal wish, but as I mentioned before, this decision is not for everyone. Sometimes a care giver can offer more and be more effective when there is some distance between them and the patient. The break may allow a better perspective and more energy to spare.

There was a time when I worried that my father would wear himself out before my mother and I knew how much he wanted to keep her at home so I told him that if anything ever happened to him first, I would take Mom into my home instead of placing her in a nursing home. But instead of the gratitude I expected, my father had me announce in the presence of my sisters that I could not promise such a thing. He had the foresight to know that we cannot always follow through on our best intentions and he did not want to me to feel guilty about an impossible decision in the future.

We all tried the best we could to share the responsibility of my mother. Once my sister thought it would be a good idea to take her to the Y for a swimming session at the pool. She seemed to like it but at one point, my sister could not see her anymore. Mom had decided to get out of the pool; she got herself half dressed, wrapped her wet suit around her wrist and walked home which is about 2 miles away through intersections and busy traffic. I still don't know how she found her way home but she did manage to arrive safely. My sister was in a panic and called the house to inform my Dad only to hear my mother's voice on the other end, innocently answering the phone.

During the most devastating final stages of her disease, Dad was constantly at her bedside, reassuring her of his presence by holding her hand, patting her hair and speaking in soft tones. He often kissed her and openly cried as he sat on the small stool by her side. Sometimes, her eyes would remain opened, other times they would stare blankly in the distance but he remained at her side and continued to share her bed every night. The day she died and was laid in her casket was the first time Dad was forced to leave her completely alone and it broke his heart.

For these reasons and many more, I dedicate my book to my Dad, my inspiration and life time hero.

Rememberance

Fifteen years is a long time to say good bye but I feel like I've made peace with my Mom. Some of the fondest memories I have are remembering her as a grandmother because once I had my own children, the role of motherhood became clear. I feel fortunate that I was given the time to appreciate that. I can picture Mom caressing babies, smiling and talking with them and in later years, making bread with them, playing in the snow and enjoying the rewards of their laughter. She once told me she wished she could have become a grandmother before becoming a mother! She was never too busy to spend time with her grandchildren and would often tell us she was always available to baby sit for us at any time. I remember once, calling her at the last minute to ask her to watch my son, Tim, for me but at the same time, wanting to be sure I was not interfering with any plans she may already have made. She reassured me that her day was wide open and that she was on her way to my home in Buckfield. It wasn't until a week later that I learned she had dropped out of a tennis match to spend time with Tim, proving that it was not only her days that were wide open for her family, but her heart as well. Mom was a born giver without expecting anything in return until the ravages of her disease finally forced her into requiring and receiving the special care, attention and support that Dad so generously and lovingly provided for her.

Near the end, there were times when she had uncontrollable shaking spells and we tried holding her to soothe them away but it was always the sound of Dad's voice and his familiar touch that had the most calming effect. I am entirely convinced that she felt his presence and loyalty until the day she died and I pray that in her own way she was also able to cherish the better years and many accomplishments of her life.

In spite of the general weakness and debilitating effects of Alzheimer's disease, I believe the most difficult times for Mom were in the beginning when she began realizing and experiencing a loss of herself. Each day would end in a collection of fragmented pieces only to be repeated the next day in varying degrees. It was during this time that I lost the mother I knew best. At the end, we lost her again, but it was more like losing a helpless child. As the disease progressed, she became more consumed and it became that much more painful for her family and friends to observe. But as difficult as it was to witness her decline there were subtle gifts in her passing; the greatest being that she was able to spend her last few days at their summer cottage in Poland, Maine, near the serenity of the lake with so many loving family members and friends dropping in to visit and share stories. It was as close to heaven as she could physically be. Another great gift is the renewal of family bonding during those intimate moments of grief.

There is also a deep sense of hope in knowing that through her family, there will be happier times with more weddings and births for generations to come.

Alzheimer's is a disease riddled with stages of irrationality, confusion, fear and finally, submission but throughout the entire process Mom was blessed with the solace of Dad's comfort and security to help her navigate a peaceful course to the bitter end, and in that, we are all blessed.

Suzanne Johnson

'Til Death Do Us Part

It's been nine days since my mother died and the knowledge of her absence is distant and surreal as I write these words. Though I do not have a clear definition of where she has gone and the sense of loss is great, her legacy lives on in the memory of my parents' love and the inner strength of soul that I treasure as her gift to me. The word 'cherish' barely defines the feelings my father has for my mother. Yet with the pain associated with her departure, I hope he can find the peace of mind he deserves with his two greatest wishes having been granted. The first, that he would outlive my mother in good health to provide the necessary care for her. The second wish was that she would remain in the comfort of her home throughout her entire illness.

Mom was one of the unfortunate victims of Alzheimer's disease, fighting a courageous and tragic battle. She was diagnosed in 1990 but had exhibited signs of confusion and disorientation for two to three years prior. Dad noticed that she had become repeatedly forgetful and was unable to carry out simple tasks such as writing out checks or putting food away and her unusual behavior finally became serious enough to warrant a neurological exam.

Alzheimer's disease is positively identified through brain pathology at the time of autopsy but a qualified neurologist is often able to diagnose the disease with over 90% accuracy through a series of specialized tests and exams, so with mixed emotions, my father reluctantly scheduled an appointment for his wife.

Following a battery of cognitive evaluations, a CAT scan and some lab work, the doctor ordered further blood work, a complete physical, and a vast array of medical tests lasting well over two hours. The results suggested the grim diagnosis of Alzheimer's disease. I remember the day that Dad gave me the news. I had gone to their home for a visit and to find out about the outcome of Mom's tests. He never said much in her presence but as I left, he walked me out to the car, rubbed his eyes and said, "It looks like your mother has Alzheimer's." The echo of those words still ominously resonates today. At that time, Alzheimer's disease was just becoming a household word with Ronald Reagan's diagnosis in 1994. I had seen it in print and had heard it spoken, but had never experienced it on a personal level. A hollow fear of the unknown gripped my heart, despite not understanding the total impact and effects of this horrific disease on the individual and their family. The progressive damage created by the physical deterioration of the body and erosion of the soul of its victims was relatively removed from my frame of experience. I would later learn through research and personal experience how Alzheimer's methodically robs the spirit and steals away precious memories and the essence of a life, while helpless family members and friends watch in pain and grief.

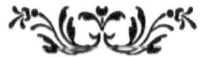

For a while, we followed the instructions of numerous doctors with their pharmaceutical trials of specialized medicine, never knowing whether the side effects would outweigh the benefits. In June of 1995, Dad was informed that there was no longer a need for Mom to see a neurologist. He handed him a year's prescription for Cognex and referred her to a general practitioner in Portland. My father was not ready to forfeit the struggle and felt he needed more answers so he decided to pursue another neurologist in the Lewiston area. At the office, I waited with Mom and Dad in the small waiting room of typical blocky chairs and outdated magazines. On the pale green wall was an abstract painting of what appeared to be two vases in the shadow of some flowers. My Dad made me laugh when he said, "Do you know what I see when I look at that picture?" I could tell we both saw the same image—the shape of a woman giving birth! Regardless of inappropriate humor, it was a relief to share a lighter moment in contrast with the continuous grim news from the doctors.

Our new doctor was pleasant but seemed far too young to have studied the many years required for a degree in neurology. His office was narrow with a white ceiling and white walls. Mom was seated directly in front of him with her hands folded, innocently smiling with her head tilted to the side, ankles crossed and slightly swinging. She seemed comfortable with him and gave the appearance of having met him before. He asked her a series of questions regarding what year it was, who the president was, asked her to spell HAND backwards and to repeat three consecutive words. She was unable to answer correctly and I wonder if she knew her answers were wrong or simply became tired of the 'game' because when he asked her to tell him her birth date, she smiled, glanced over at Dad and said, "You tell him."

The saddest stage of Mom's disease was when she reached the point of realizing she was losing herself. Questioning reality must be the most overwhelming personal fear. She once admitted to Dad, "I don't like the way I think" and "I don't know what the matter is." At night, she would wake up and go looking for her father who had passed away in 1986 and would often refer to my father as 'her Daddy' as opposed to addressing him as her husband, Ray. She would walk out of the house not knowing where she was, prompting Dad to place dead bolts on all the doors and hiding the car keys. She could not complete simple tasks anymore and would leave the water running, forget to close doors and put inappropriate items in the freezer. Her moods would vacillate from confusion to frustration but the anger that is so common with Alzheimer's was nonexistent in Mom. I attribute that fact to my father's insight and sensitivity towards her needs. She could feel the comfort of his love and his endless patience so the urge to become angry or defensive was diffused. Part of it may also have been her demeanor but we were fortunate not to have witnessed the symptoms of angry bitterness and betrayal.

Following restless nights of erratic sleep, Mom would often be confused first thing in the morning. Dad would play familiar music that would seem to make her happy and even feel like dancing. This became a routine and set the tone for the morning. Once in a while I would get her to play ping-pong with me in the basement. It was so easy to make her laugh by sending a wild serve or performing silly antics. I did not realize at the time how much I would miss the sound of that laughter.

Over time, Dad learned the importance of being tactful in his approach when Mom was irrational because she would become frustrated and more confused from not knowing how to correct her mistakes. During the very early stage when trips to Florida were still manageable, my husband and two young children flew down from Maine to visit. We took a ride to a nearby beach, parked the car and walked about 500 feet towards the ocean. Dad suddenly remembered he had forgotten his sunglasses in the car and was about to turn around to retrieve them when Mom said she would go instead. She was still aware enough to know Dad had been suffering from worn cartilage in both knees and extended walking was painful for him. In retrospect, I should have offered to go with her, but at the time she seemed coherent enough to find her way. Minutes later, she came running from the opposite end of the beach in tears, saying she had gotten lost. Dad held her close until she was able to regain her composure, but we were all quite shaken by this frightening turn of events.

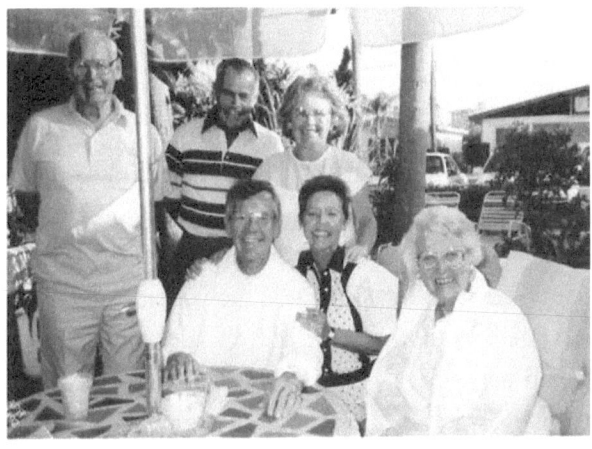

Having a great time in Florida with friends and relatives. 1992

Alzheimer's disease has a cruel way of being undetectable to a certain extent and it's victims may appear to be functioning normally. From the outside, a person suffering from the early stages may look quite healthy, carry on conversations, go out to eat, enjoy music and dancing while at the same time, be completely dependent upon a spouse or care giver for safety, stability and survival. They can even display the characteristics of a contented, well-adjusted individual who is at peace with the world while the underlying turmoil of one who can no longer even recognize his/her own family is hidden from view. Many distant friends and relations never come close to understanding what the primary care giver experiences and at times can even diminish the gravity of the situation. To an outsider it was difficult to see beyond Mom's neatly dressed and well-cared for appearance due to my father's attention. The irreversible dementia, memory loss, constant repetitions and heartbreak were always discreetly concealed.

In 1993, Dad required surgery on his knees. This meant someone staying with Mom and shuttling her to the hospital and back. She would ask where her 'Daddy' was, and we would take her to the hospital but no sooner had we left, she would again ask where her 'Daddy' was. At times while Dad was in the hospital she became disturbed with a sense of alienation. Before surgery and anticipating the problem Dad had made a tape recording of his voice. All we needed to do was play his voice for Mom when we felt she needed reassurance. We used it a few times and it seemed to console her for a brief moment but she would soon forget she had heard his voice and become worried again, so I tried to occupy her thoughts by encouraging her to start knitting to pass the time. I was amazed at how her nimble fingers could so easily maneuver the colorful yarn and needles. Everywhere we went, we carried along her knitting bag so she could work on her 'scarf' that eventually measured over 15 feet long! Dad's recovery from surgery was quick and he was soon in charge of caring for Mom again, but even under his watchful eye, she would find ways to cause concern. Once she had locked herself out of the house while taking clothes off the line from the back porch and was found on the front porch with no idea of how she had gotten there. Another time, Dad had mysteriously found a partially burnt stuffed animal on the vanity in the bathroom that had burned enough to blacken the Formica top.

By August of 1995, Dad decided that it was time for Mom to have a Personal Care Assistant (PCA). We found Doris. Mom's coordination and ability to focus was declining and having another person involved with her care became necessary. The timing was such that she was still able to get to know Doris and acquire her trust. Doris remained with us for nine years and became a very loyal part of the family. We all tried to keep a normal semblance of order to Mom's life by preserving her routines as best as we could. Small things like reaching for the tube of toothpaste first, then the brush, or putting her right arm in her coat sleeve first, etc., seemed to alleviate some confusion by allowing her to retain a familiar process. When she would come to my home to visit with Dad, it never mattered whether the ground was wet or dry, she would always wipe her shoes on my welcome mat before entering the house; force of habit; something familiar.

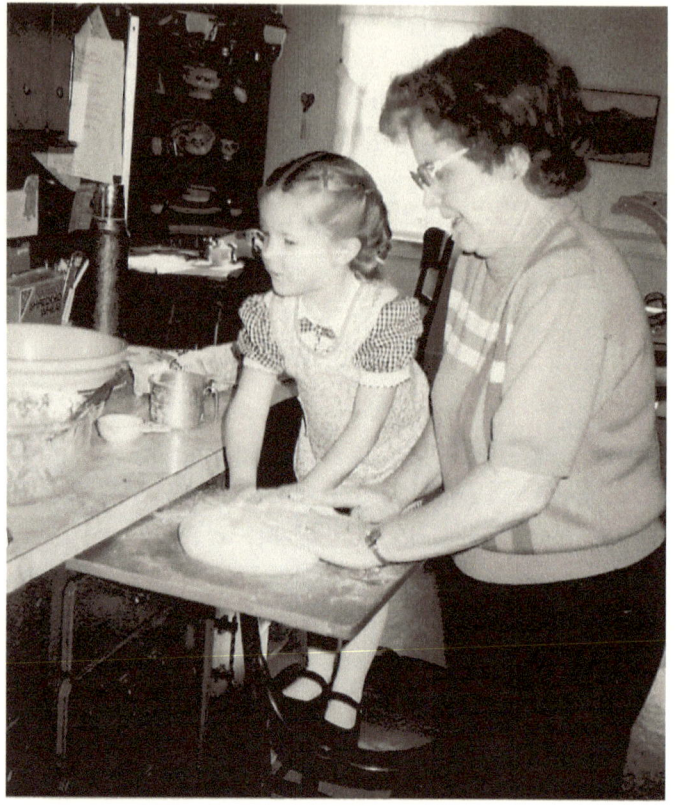

Bea and granddaughter Emily baking bread. 1988

Yet in spite of her increasing dementia, Mom was always willing to help with chores around the house. She was physically fit, strong for her years and had always enjoyed working hard. One afternoon at the lake, while she was sweeping the porch steps, she fell forward onto the walkway. Dad noticed her lying on the ground and ran to her aid. She was conscious but unable to tell Dad what had happened. He rushed her to the Poland Emergency Clinic where they were unable to determine any injuries so they returned to camp and she helped Dad finish mowing the lawn!

Two days later, they were back at camp raking leaves and hauling them away on a tarpaulin mat, but later that evening, Mom appeared to be sore and was having difficulty walking but could not communicate her discomfort. Another visit to the Medical Center revealed a pulled muscle in her groin that finally responded well to heat treatments after 14 days. Yet throughout the entire ordeal, Mom was cooperative, kept up a good disposition and never complained.

It was beginning to become more difficult to decipher Mom's emotions. Her speech was limited and she rarely cried so when she felt sick or accidentally fell down, we had to rely on guess work to evaluate her particular situation. Often times, the signs were not always evident. There was a time when Mom appeared a little more quiet than usual but exhibited no other symptoms of malaise. The next morning, Dad was unable to rouse her or get her attention. She appeared to be in a trance like state. The ambulance was called and tests were done to reveal an intestinal infection, slight dehydration and a yeast infection. Living with Alzheimer's must cause the victim to feel trapped within the most bizarre condition. I would have been curious to know what was inside her mind at times just to get a perspective of what her world was really like. There were days when Doris would come over and Mom would ignore her. She would have nothing to do with her at all. This uncharacteristic behavior was unusual and I wonder if she could have resented the idea of having to need assistance or if it was just a symptom of her disease. There are still so many frustrating and perplexing questions that will forever remain unanswered.

As time wore on, Mom began to have more mood swings and would sleep longer hours. She lost interest in simple chores like making the bed, ironing clothes, cross stitching and knitting but never lost her appreciation for what Dad could do for her. He was such a huge part of her heart. Her spirit would lighten when he entered the room and his eyes would search for her as well. She often told him he was a "good Dad" and he would thrive for that simple reward. It was the beginning of a new relationship that would keep them always together yet forever apart. This dedicated commitment towards each other was steadfast and would survive the test of brutal time.

Two weeks before Christmas of 1995, when the ground was covered with snow, Mom (at 72 years old) was outside shoveling the walkway with Dad. Later that afternoon, the family came to decorate the Christmas tree. Dad played some holiday music and we all danced in the living room but the frivolity was overshadowed by hearing my mother sing 'Silent Night' over my shoulder as I played the piano. She sung the familiar lyrics so naturally but could not formulate her own words into a complete thought, and although she did enjoy herself to the fullest that night she had absolutely no recollection of it the next day.

Holidays and special events were beginning to have sad undertones. They would force us to project what the next holiday would be like and consequently make us feel thankful for the moment and grateful for the better memories of the past. It was fortunate that my sisters and I were able to convince Dad to make plans for a 50th anniversary celebration in March. At first he believed it was too much trouble, then maybe too difficult for Mom to enjoy with all the uncertainties of her life but finally, after some gentle, subtle coaxing, he gave in, allowing the event to proceed.

Mom looked so elegant that day wearing a pale pink skirt and jacket with off white trim, gold buttons, white sandals and of course, her radiant smile. She danced to the music, assisted Dad in cutting the cake and seemed to enjoy the crowd even though it was obvious that she had no idea that the party was in her honor. There was a time when I had to keep her from refolding the napkins on the tables but she was easily redirected to the dance floor. When it came time for my cousin to propose a very tender and sentimental toast, there was not a dry eye in the room except for my Mom who was casually eating peanuts out of a candy bowl, captured in a bittersweet moment of time.

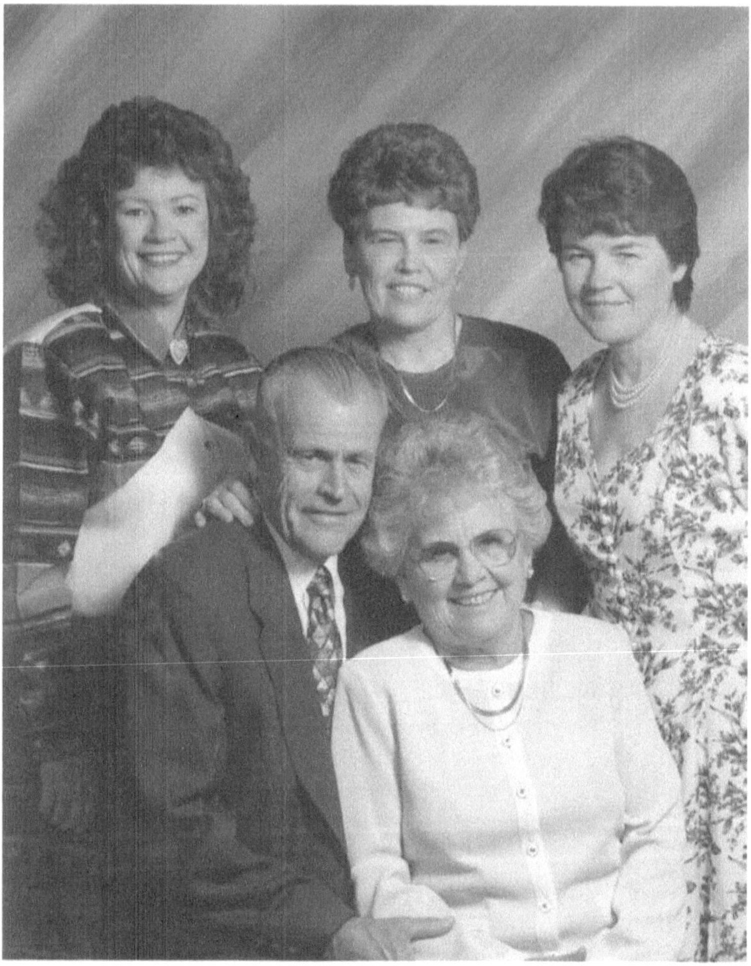

Fiftieth wedding anniversary 1995. (left to right, back row to front)
Elaine, Anita, Sue, Dad and Mom

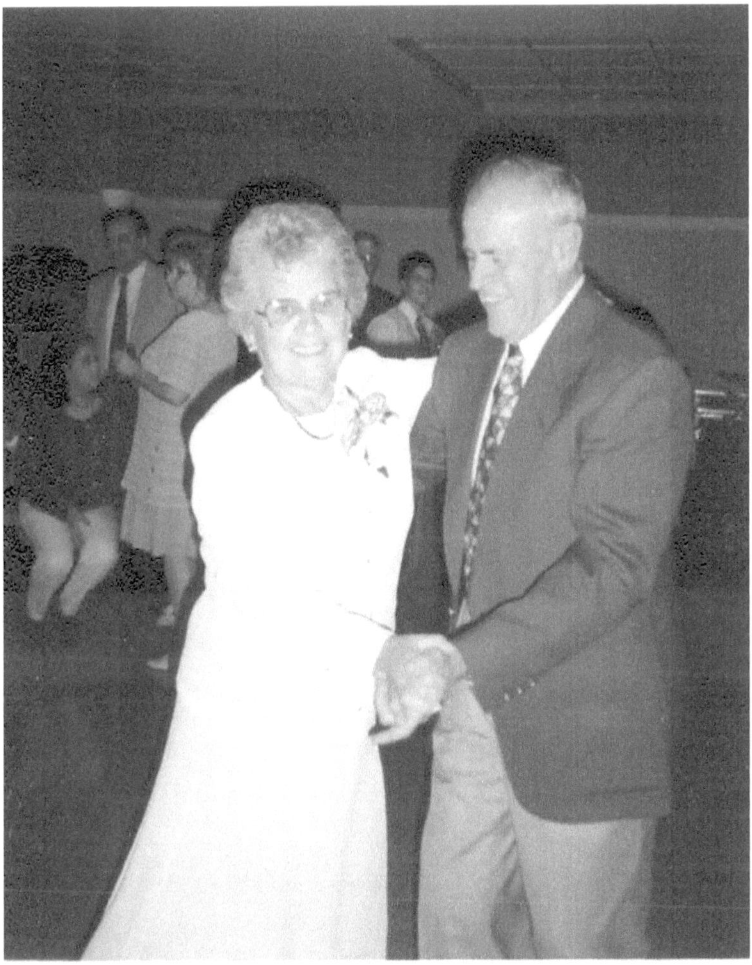

Dancing to the music at 50th anniversary party.

In mid-winter, Mom and Dad were still able to travel to Florida for a few weeks. Their condo was situated on the beach with a full view of spectacular sunsets over the ocean. They enjoyed walking the beach, going out to dinner with friends and hitting a few golf balls but if they tried to do too much for one day, Mom would become overtired and this would aggravate her confusion. She was still taking Cognex which seemed to delay the inevitable but it wasn't enough to prevent her from being too ill to take many more trips down south.

In the spring of 1996, she had another appointment with the same neurologist in Lewiston who noticed increased deterioration. She was beginning to have accidents with her bowels and wore special undergarments. She also seemed to become more dependent on Dad and would worry when he was not around. As soon as he was out of her sight, she would ask for him and wonder where he was in spite of repeatedly having been told. One day at camp after Dad had left for errands, she asked me where "her Daddy" had gone. I told her he was away for a short while and he would be right back. She turned to me with the most sorrowful look and said, "Don't lie to me." I was wearing sunglasses at the time and I pulled them off so she could look into my eyes and told her that I would not lie to her. She slowly looked down, shook her head in confusion and I feel that we both cried inside from exasperation.

On happier days, I could keep her occupied by taking walks or working on simple projects with her. We carved pumpkins, baked cookies, made puzzles, played checkers, did some drawing, folded clothes, played tennis, went swimming, played whiffle ball, and even went skating and cross country skiing. One warm summer afternoon in particular, we took a ride in the paddle boat and called Dad on his cell phone from out on the lake. She was always willing to try new things and enjoyed a good time.

It was around this time that Dad would have Mom write a line or two a day in a notebook to practice her writing skills. Each day she would write a sentence pertaining to what she had done or a feeling she had and sign her name. Some days she needed more guidance than others but upon viewing the words she wrote, the notable decline was obvious until there finally came a day when she could no longer write or even remember how to hold a pen.

The following pages clearly illustrate these changes.

7-7-95 — Big Brother ~~Big~~ Bill came today
FRI Beatrice Legendre

7-11-95 — Tim Hellted Me Play Tennis —
We Had A Good Time eg
Beatrice Legendre

7-19-95 It was bod? Birthday Sunday
8:20 AM Beatrice Legendre

7-30-95 Went to Cherrd Today
church
Beatrice Legendre

8-3-95 UE went to the animal farm today
Beatrice Legendre

8-11-95 I drove the car today
Beatrice Legendre

8-22-95 I am going to have my Harir done today
Beatrice Legendre

8-28-95 Beatrice Legendre
We moned The Lawen today

9-9-95 Beatrice Legendre
SAT I cooked the Bacon today

9-16-95 B We went to indian Pond today
Beatrice Legendre

10-31-95
TUES Myr Fegirs Bettertoday
      Beatrice Legendre

11-15-95 Mecwent To Borthand Today
WED Beatrice Legendre

11-22-95 Beatrice Legendre Xmas-Tree to day
Wed-

12-10-95 Vetrim Legendre Xmas-Tree to day
SUN Beatrice Legendre

2-1-96 UE went to Whedoctor to day
THURS Beatrice Legendre

2-15-96 I Rode the Bike
        Beatrice Legendre

3-9-96 Viw fwent Bowlingito day
        Beatrice Legendre

4-2-96 Bill and Lawra Came Todo Aw
TUES Bell Beatrice Legendre
      Beatrice Legendre

6-4-96 Bea Beatrice Leg Legendre
TUES Ule Bik w

9-5-96 Beatrice Legendre

11/4/96 Beatr BBL LLla aw

Mom was beginning to have more difficulty in dressing herself. She seemed to be able to manage if her clothes were handed to her, one item at a time but she would sometimes apply layer upon layer of clothing and had difficulty finding the arm holes. One morning Dad found her sitting on the side of her bed with her pants on and trying to pull panty hose up over them. Such a disheartening sight but Dad would gently assist her and tell her she was doing well and that he loved her while another small piece of his heart would break. Throughout my childhood years, I had never really noticed many outward expressions of love between my parents but during these times, Dad had become very demonstrative with his feelings towards his wife. He always held and patted her hand when they were together and often kissed her, calling her "his Darling" or "my Honey" and frequently commented on how beautiful she was or on the soft outline of her profile and striking blue eyes.

One morning at home, Mom had forgotten to do something Dad had asked her to do and he jokingly said to her, "You don't listen to me, Bea" She looked up at him and replied, "I'm sorry". It made my father cry to tell me about this. He said he would never say anything like that to her again and blamed himself for his 'insensitivity' but the most sorrowful grievance was Mom's incapacity to console him.

In October 1996, Mom developed what appeared to be neurological spasms, accompanied with a sudden shout. It was like a jolt of lightening that could send her to the floor. They would vary in intensity but were always very frightening. The fact that she never broke any bones or suffered any serious injury with the falls she took over the years was probably because she had always taken such good care of herself by staying active and eating well. She had also taken such pride in her healthy and perfectly white teeth but her ruthless disease had cast yet another insult by limiting the care she could give them, and inadvertently, allowing them to turn yellow and begin to fall out as she neared the end.

Short term memory was progressively failing now and she began to find pleasure in small things such as dolls, stuffed animals and looking through her jewelry box. She was especially attracted to the glittery pieces and would spend a large amount of time carefully sorting through her collection, totally enthralled with her task. There were times when we could laugh along with her but I wish I could have enjoyed her more as a whole person in her older years so that I could have shared the joys of motherhood with her. I saved a post card she had sent her grandchildren from Florida because she had signed it 'From Aunt Bea and Uncle Ray.' The eminent progression of a downward spiral was evident. My son was eight and my daughter was four when my Mother began experiencing behavioral changes. Yet the care and nurturing she had so generously given to both my children when they were younger was instilled in their hearts so that the memory as a loving grandmother overpowered the image of the disease. I do feel thankful for that.

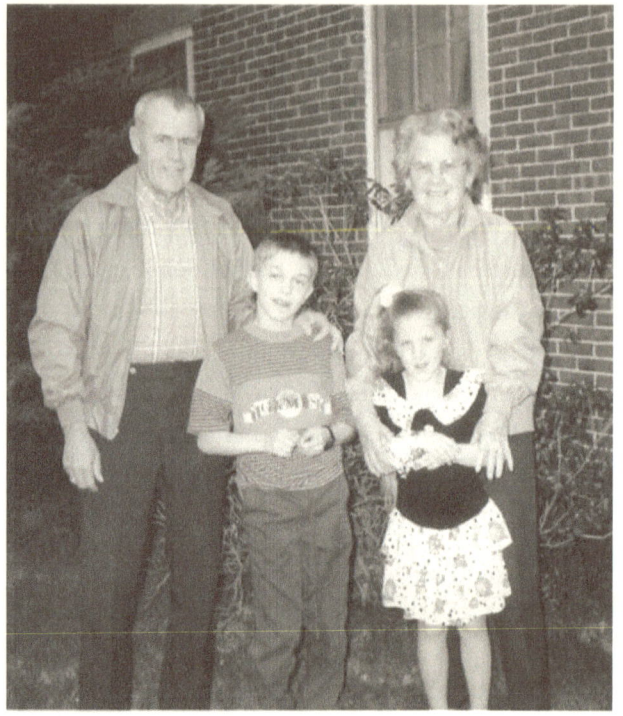

Ray and Bea with grandchildren Tim and Emily.

In January of 1997, Mom was taken off Cognex because the side effects had a chance of causing more damage than the benefits. Without the Cognex she appeared to be more confused and quiet, especially in the mornings and did not seem to be as cheerful. Her coordination had worsened and she was walking very slowly, so with renewed hope, she was placed on Aricept. Within two weeks, Dad noticed some improvement but at this point, we were grasping at straws. She was still able to get out of bed by herself but needed total hygienic care. She would remember how to wash her hands if she saw someone else doing the same thing and could wipe her hands on the other end of the towel. Her bed making skills were waning but she could still feed herself and responded well to music. Dad would hold her hands while the music played and she would rhythmically bounce to the sound. It was a familiar and joyful routine while it lasted but was soon to become another stolen pleasure.

Life became more unpredictable as far as activities and daily planning. Some days Mom could greet Dad with a cheerful 'Hi' in the morning, make the bed up, put her glasses on and be ready for breakfast, while other times she would sleep very late and wake up with not even enough energy to brush her teeth so daily scheduling was sporadic. Yet in spite of her mental challenge, Mom maintained a strong will and was eager to please. She sought recognition and approval from the one who mattered most in her life, and Dad was always there to make sure her efforts were validated. He somehow found the strength to curb his frustrations and foster the encouragement needed to grant her the quality of life she so well deserved and in return, he received the occasional acknowledgement of her grateful love by a certain look from the past that made him feel complete. One evening while they were out for supper, Dad casually asked her if she loved him and she answered, "Of course I love you." It had been a long time since he had heard her use those words and the impact was profound! He was sadly learning to savor precious memories and appreciate the few simple joys.

In November of 1997, Mom weighed 158 pounds (on a 5′ 4″ frame). The doctor thought she might have a thyroid problem or that her blood sugar level might be abnormal. We watched her diet and tried to get her to exercise more but the weight remained the same. Had we known that she would melt down to 70 pounds at the end, we might not have worried as much.

Alzheimer's disease is an affliction of constant losses in varying degrees. Mom was now losing the dexterity in her hands and fingers. She could no longer sew buttons, cut up her food or cross stitch pillow cases anymore. Realizing she could no longer sew was especially difficult to accept because there had been a certain peace in watching her work with a needle and thread. It offered us a brief interlude into how her life used to be along with the many other skills she had mastered that were no longer within her reach. I wonder how much awareness a patient actually comprehends about his/her demise. I would hope the disease would at least have the mercy to spare its victims the torment of despair.

Neurological spasms continued to occur in varying strengths and frequency without any explanation. An EEG had been done to no avail and it was simply a matter of her being lucky if they occurred while she was safely seated. There was no forewarning. One day at camp, she was seated at the picnic table when a strong spasm sent her reeling backwards, hitting her head on the ground as her knees grazed the underneath of the table. She expressed the element of surprise, but did not seem to be hurt.

Mom was slowly going downhill by February 1998. Her attention span was short and selective. She was still able to attend a few family functions etc, but it was the young children and the babies in the crowd that captivated her. If she was at a supermarket or mall, she would walk right up to infants in carts to touch and play with them. Most young mothers understood after Dad explained the situation but there were others who remained understandably wary.

Mom's auditory sense was another area of concern around this time. Dad would call out her name and she would walk faster in the opposite direction, seemingly not knowing where his voice was coming from. Crowds were also making her more tired and confused. In the summer of 98, a foundry outing was held at their camp on Thompson Lake with much activity and commotion. She became alarmed and frustrated when it was time to move from one place to another. People tried to help but she became more confused and upset. She settled when the crowd dispersed. A similar incident occurred while we were leaving the theater one night. At the end of the show, the audience had to exit off of a staircase. Mom stood at the top of the stairs and froze. People were waiting to get past but she would not budge. Often times when Alzheimer patients need to step down or over an uneven pathway, they perceive it as a darkened abyss and become gripped with fear. Dad's technique was to gently talk her through this fear without making her feel as though she was being pulled forward into a bottomless pit, but well-meaning people tried putting their hands on her to guide her down and she would not move. We finally let everyone go by, then Dad was free to take his time, regain her confidence and reach her comfort zone.

On good days, Mom enjoyed taking walks outdoors but her gait had begun to change. She had more of a shuffle to her step and was becoming unsteady but she still liked being outdoors and 'helping' with chores. On a beautiful October afternoon, Dad and Mom had taken a ride out to camp to rake leaves. Dad raked and Mom tried to help but it was more like following him around the yard. At one point, she wandered over to the picnic table and noticed a small yellow leaf that had fallen off a tree onto the table. She picked it up and carried it to Dad, handing it over as if to say, "This is for you." The tenderness of this gesture brought Dad to tears and to this day, that leaf remains on the refrigerator where he had taped it on that memorable afternoon.

By the beginning of the new year of 1999, Mom needed help to finish her meals but along with her decline came a few treasured blessings. She would still utter "I love you" to my Dad, either in response to him or during a time when he was attending to her needs. One night, as they laid in bed at the end of another long day, she placed her hand on his cheek and gently patted his face as if to indicate in her own way that she understood how complicated their lives had become.

Daily routines were scheduled around Mom's needs, making Dad's plans uncertain and spontaneous but it was clear that she would always be the priority in his life. He always spoke to her with endearing tones and never lost his patience with any tasks, no matter how difficult or taxing and did his best to preserve her dignity with a semblance of normality. There were always beautiful bouquets with hand written love notes on the table for every birthday and anniversary, and although the flowers would wither and the messages remained unread their meanings were never unspoken.

Traveling became more of a chore because Mom was apprehensive about getting into the car. She could not seem to coordinate her actions necessary to stoop down and sit in the passenger seat. She could walk up to the opened door, but once within arm's reach, she would place her hands on the door frame, and be unwilling to maneuver herself any further, so when Dad traded his car, he purchased a Dodge Durango that was more spacious and easier for her to step up into, although it wasn't long before he had to adapt a step stool for her to climb up onto. Selling his car was a major turning point for Dad because it signified more changes in their lives. On the day he sold it, he was up in the middle of the night, staring into the vacant space in his garage, silently weeping for the past.

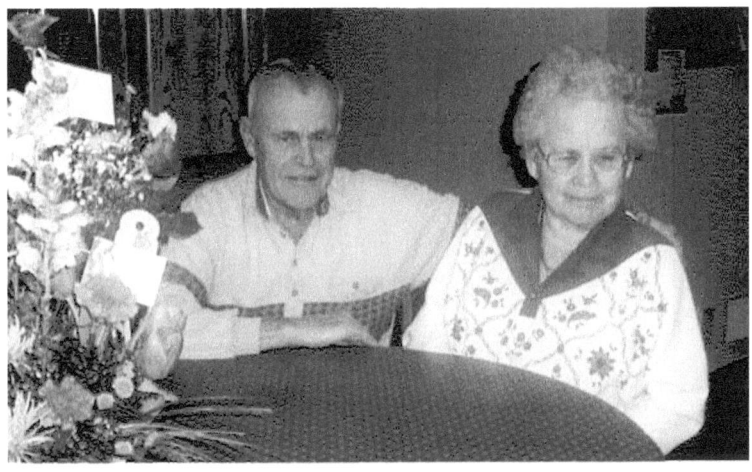

Fifty sixth anniversary bouquet. 2001 Ray and Bea.

On March 28 1999, Dad noted:

This morning, I realized that she had not said her little phrase of 'You are a good Dad.' This really hurts because it was probably her last words to me. I was upset all morning, just thinking about this.

It was also about this time that she was unable to tolerate long walks anymore. Her gait had a quickening shuffle-like quality with a tendency to lean forward and at times would walk past the house, needing redirection to turn onto the walkway. The disease was becoming a continuous progression of firsts and lasts. We were beginning to marvel at any limited sense of observation. One morning, she looked out at the rain and said. "Lots of water!" Even slight verbal exclamations became pertinent to us and worthy to share with each other. I once tried to have her say, "Hi Sue" and when she repeated "Hoo Hoo," I was thrilled!

Her spasms were still occurring at intervals and becoming strong enough to knock her to the ground even from a sitting position. Surprisingly, she never seriously injured herself, which would have compounded the amount of care she already required. Her level of alertness would vary throughout the day and Dad became accustomed to intermittent periods of lucidity, always finding his greatest rewards in her gracious smile and her soft touch.

Evenings, in the summer of '99 were commonly spent in the swing at camp, watching the sunset on the lake. Dad would sing "Let me call you Sweetheart" and she would seem to recognize the melody and even try to hum along, oblivious to anyone but Dad. Yet once again, as time wore on, her coordination worsened making it nearly impossible for her to get on or off the swing and this sweet reverie would also have to end as her very life would, within the next five years.

We all knew the end would come, but we were never sure in what form. One night in January, I had a dream about Mom dying. Someone (presumably Dad) had to follow her and there was some chaotic discussion about an injection for euthanasia. I asked how long it took and a nurse said it only took 10 seconds but many people panic after eight and want to come back but cannot. I was in a small room with a window. I can envision only Dad's face through the glass. He was lying down and had been injected. I am now near his bed and I hold him as I count to myself. I'm telling him how much I love him and by eight seconds, he tells me he can see her. He is calm and I see her too, only I see her in his mind. She is smiling and perfectly well. I tell him to tell her I love her too, and he leaves …

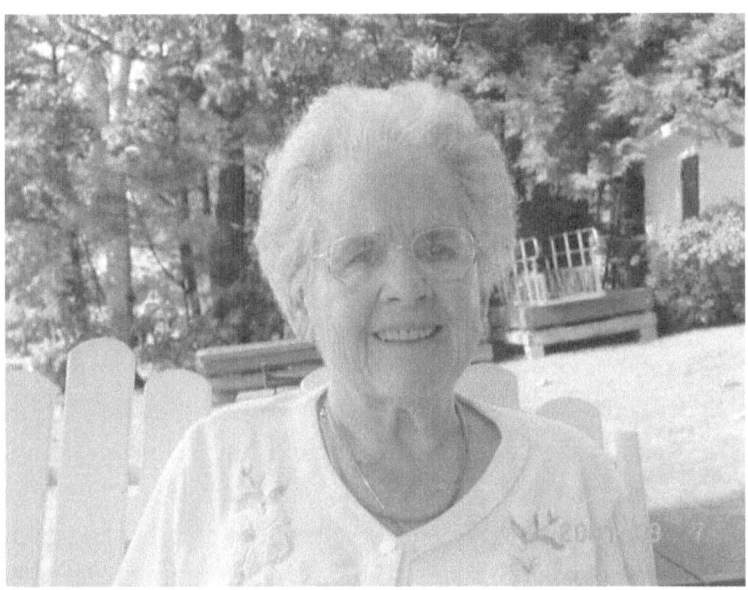

Peaceful summer day in the swing at camp. *"Let Me Call You Sweetheart" August 1999.*

Mom's balance began to waver in the fall of 1999 and she would tend to lean towards her right side while seated, sometimes needing to be propped with a pillow. She could still feed herself but needed occasional assistance with utensils, although within a few short months, she required more help. Her needs were increasing and along with the changes, her emotions began to falter. It was evident that she frequently recognized Dad when he spoke to her. On good days, she would make eye contact and smile at him with a slight characteristic nod of her head acknowledging him with sweet remembrance. This usually brought grateful tears to his eyes and consoled him for lonelier days when all she could provide was a blank stare. Dad had also noticed that it had been months since he had last seen her cry.

Mom weighed 146 pounds at the beginning of 2000. Her appetite was fair but she seemed to lack taste receptors. Her favorite foods meant nothing and she could chew bitter vitamin pills with no reaction and would often hold food or fluids in her mouth, sometimes, without anyone noticing. I took her shopping one morning after having brushed her teeth following breakfast. We were driving in my car when she noticed a baby in a stroller. She started to smile and the foamy toothpaste water from her mouth came pouring out.

Mom's gait had a more noticeable shuffle and her pace was slowing down. Dad would never let go of her hand for fear that she would wander in the wrong direction or lose her balance, but for those who did not know the elderly couple, they portrayed the triumph of everlasting love.

Gradually, Mom became physically weaker and was having more trouble going down stairs. She could hardly take walks anymore and spent many hours dozing during the day. There were times when she would sleep most of the day, but become more alert in the evenings. "Sun downing" in Alzheimer's often occurs as a symptom of the disease. It causes tension, irritability, phobic tendencies, restlessness, hallucinations, fear and for some reason, is usually associated with dusk. Perhaps the onset of darkness has an ominous effect on those already living in the dark. Many patients need medication in the evenings to curb the anxiety, but Mom frequently would perk up at this time of day. There were days when she could have slept through her meals with little response while awake, and then be ready to smile, focus her eyes on those around her by five o'clock in the afternoon and her long day of unconsciousness would give way to a welcomed break in the clouds.

Dad was still bringing Mom to church on Saturday afternoons. He never liked attending any sort of function without her and if it was not feasible for Mom to attend, he would deny himself the opportunity as well. Mom had lost most of her ability to communicate at this point but was still understandable in other ways. At church one evening when the sermon droned on far beyond its point, Mom tilted her head back and produced a very loud, gratifying yawn! Dad was amusingly embarrassed but later on it became too tiring for her to attend, so they both stayed home. It was strange for my Dad not to attend church after so many years of being a devout Catholic but his special situation had transformed his very life into an even more meaningful prayer.

Mom had regressed to childlike qualities but had not abandoned her need to nurture. On good nights, she would lay in bed smiling and looking directly at my Dad. She often would pat his chest and shoulder, then try to adjust the collar of his pajamas with hands as soft as an angels. Following one of these moments, Dad wrote in his journal,

She is a sweet girl.

In September 2000, Mom was very unsteady on her feet, she was beginning to drool, was dysphasic and her weight had dropped to 138 pounds. Aricept was increased to twice a day without much hope. Her disease had descended to the latter stages and the burden was heavy. We had to brace ourselves for more losses and shortly after Dad's birthday in October, Mom had to partially depend on a wheelchair for mobility.

The new year of 2001 brought on bouts with shingles, an infected toe, dryness of the eyes and unexplained bruising but Mom did not seem to experience discomfort. Even after her

intermittent falls, she would look surprised but never react in pain. Instead, she would smile at whoever was around to help re-establish herself. It's possible that the emotional and pain receptors in the affected portion of her brain had become dull allowing her at least some reprieve from her withering illness. I suppose we could consider this an extremely minor consolation because she was spared the grief of her brother's death that summer from being unaware of the event, lost in her silent world of oblivion.

There were times when Mom would not wake up in the morning and even when she would slightly rouse, she would remain in a semi-conscious state. Dad would become so alarmed and worried, repeating that he couldn't understand what was happening to her or the reason for the change. He would often blame himself for not having given her enough fluids or putting her to bed too late, or maybe she had the flu etc., constantly denying the inevitable and remaining adamant regarding circumstances that he could still control. In December, he purchased a van with a wheelchair ramp adaptation so that Mom would not be housebound. The van worked beautifully with an elevator lift in the garage. They were still able to travel together on short trips, mostly to and from the lake. He had removed the front passenger seat to install a special wheelchair lock in its place so he could simply roll her up onto the lift and fasten her chair into the space but one of the first times he had tried it, the lock was not secured and as he drove forward, her chair rolled to the back of the van, sadly emphasizing her total helplessness.

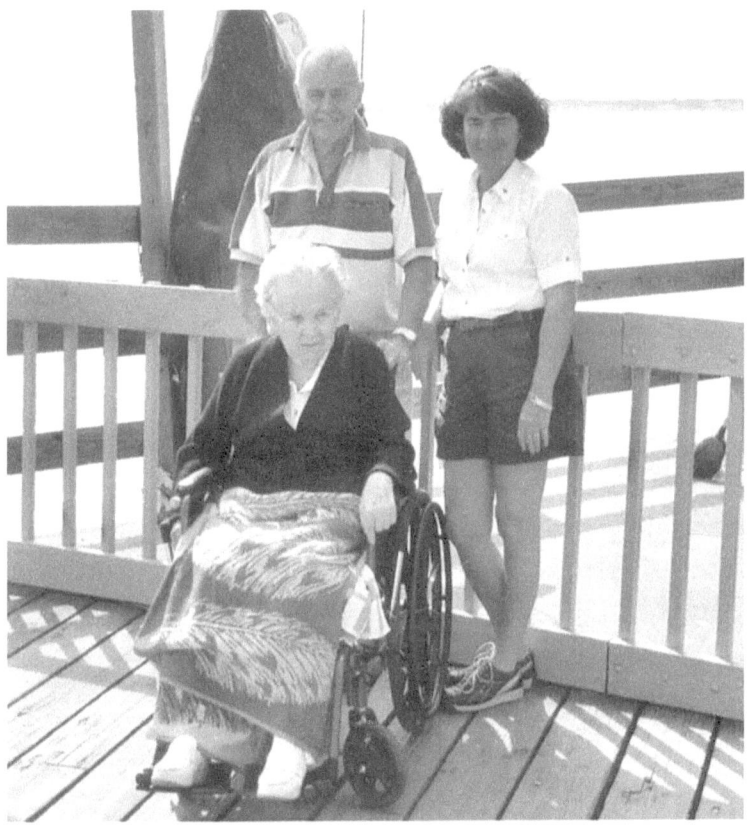

Mom, Dad and Sue at Old Orchard Beach 1999.

Mom could not speak anymore but she would still communicate with her eyes and facial expressions. Dad's voice soothed her and she would often reach out for him with a waving sort of motion. I walked in on them once when they were both sound asleep, in their separate chairs. Mom had her right hand near her heart and with her other hand, she was holding Dad's. Their heads leaned towards each other in perfect unison and for a brief moment, I wished it could have ended here, yet I knew in my heart I was selfishly not prepared to lose them both.

Mom was sleeping for longer periods these days, much to Dad's dismay. He once stated, "There will come a time when those eyes will be closed forever and I want to be able to look at them for as long as I can."

The downward spiral continued as Mom became more lethargic and despondent. Lucid moments were treasured and became rarer but it was clear that tougher times were ahead. Two people were needed to transfer her from her chair to the bed, although Dad managed to do it himself when they were alone. His body mechanics and coordinated movements were perfectly synchronized to accommodate Mom's limitations. They had always been a team in health and would be in sickness as well.

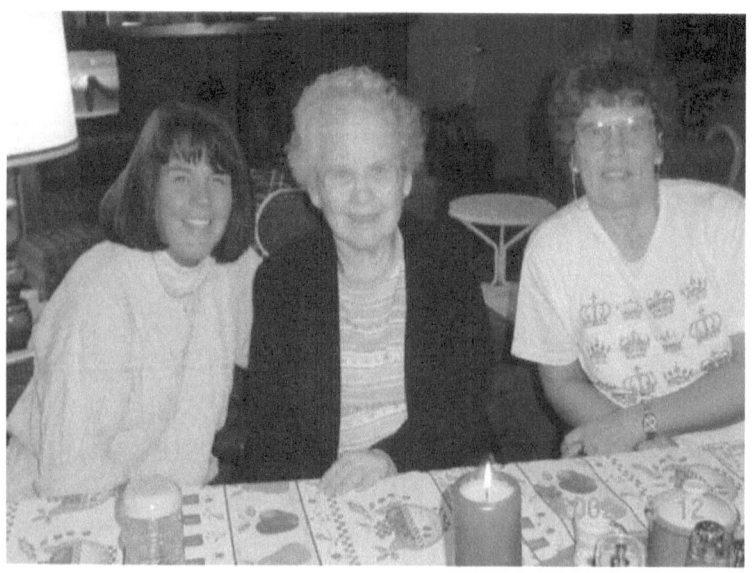

Happy February birthdays! Sue, Mom and Anita, 2002.

In January 2003 Mom began experiencing uncontrollable tremors that would generally occur upon being repositioned, or getting her in and out of bed. Her upper body would shake uncontrollably for several seconds, her pulse would race, then she would relax but seemed exhausted following each spell. It was very similar to having a seizure. As we were all going through the process with her, we gradually became accustomed to the symptoms affiliated with her disease, but it has only been since I started to write my mother's story that the devastation of her changing condition became so much more apparent and tragic in my mind.

The days, weeks and months wore on with the knowledge that in spite of the overwhelming hardships of the present, it would always be better than what the future held. Mom started to detach herself from her environment and seemed more isolated in her own world. Her muscles had atrophied and were beginning to contract. We kept a small foam ball inside her left hand to keep her fingers from curling, her head had a tendency to turn towards the left and her general muscle tone was poor. It took over an hour to feed her and she could only tolerate small sips and soft foods. There were days when she would hardly eat at all. She was weak, listless and weighed 127 pounds, but still managed to smile for Dad when he tried to gently persuade her into swallowing. She was surviving for his sake and it was as if she felt he wasn't ready to be without her yet and was going to hang on until the time was right.

In October of 2003, Mom developed what appeared to be a small cyst at the end of her spine from malnutrition and spending extended time in bed. Dad ordered a lift chair to facilitate getting her up and they would sit together in the parlor, facing the large picture window. Along the side wall hung a portrait of themselves painted during their first vacation to Florida. They had just returned from their trip when Dad told us they had purchased some 'art' work but wasn't sure how valuable it was. My sisters and I were in suspense because Dad had never indicated he had any interest in 'art' but we understood when he unveiled the oil painting and saw a beautifully-framed 18 by 24 inch portrait of the two of them wearing soft pastels. At the time, he never realized how priceless this piece of art would become because it remained one of the few things that could stir a response from Mom. As she sat in the parlor, her eyes would sometimes wander and eventually rest on the picture, causing her to smile and say, "Ooooooh."

By November of 2003, the Home Health Agency became involved in Mom's care due to the spinal cyst that would not heal. Nurses would visit to offer supportive care and apply a clean dressing twice a week.

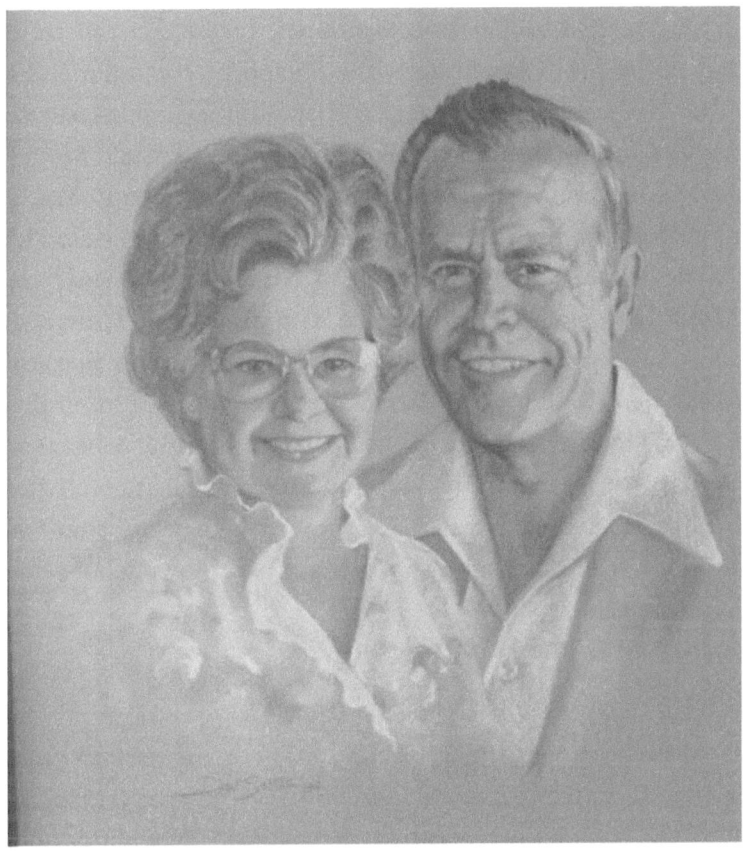

The oil painting of Bea and Ray purchased on their first trip to Florida.

We gathered for Thanksgiving Day in solemn celebration, knowing in our hearts that holidays as a complete family were becoming scarce. Mom was very tired so we put her down on the sofa to rest but she never seemed ready to wake up and join us at the table. It was another terrible first of not having her with us and the empty place setting next to Dad was even more vacant in his heart. He quietly ate his meal then sat next to her on the sofa to watch her sleep.

The next morning around noon, I received a call from Dad saying Mom would not wake up and he could not feel a pulse. My husband and I raced to Lewiston to find the Home Health nurse at Mom's side taking her blood pressure. Mom's respirations were shallow; she was perspiring and had a frantic look on her face. Dad was visibly shaken and stated he had never seen her this way. The nurse tried to ease his anxiety by saying it could be due to the fact that Mom was seeing an unfamiliar face and that she had to stretch her arm to take her blood pressure but as I observed my Mom in this frenzied state, I realized Dad had every right to be concerned because I believe Mom had just suffered a small stroke. Later that day, the left side of her face showed evidence of paralysis and she was having slightly more trouble swallowing.

Mom's last Christmas was in 2003. For the past 25 years or so, the family gathered for Christmas at a restaurant to celebrate, have dinner, and the young cousins would put on a short skit. After the performance, one of the uncles took turns each year being 'Santa' in the tailor made red velvet suit Mom had painstakingly made for the occasion back in 1976. It was enjoyable to watch the children sing and act, but when they outgrew their yearning to perform, we simply gathered for a holiday meal. For the last two years, we took Mom to the restaurant in a wheelchair and had to leave early because she would fall asleep in her chair, yet Dad always had her beautifully dressed in holiday attire with her hair freshly styled. Her relentless disease may have stripped away many of her attributes but Dad still managed to preserve her dignity to her final days. By 2003, it was too much for Mom to be awake for long periods so we all agreed to quietly celebrate Christmas at Dad's house and invited relatives to drop by afterwards. For me, this resulted in a most meaningful Christmas in that everyone expressed in a most caring way, the faithful commitment of family.

Three months after Christmas, hospice care was arranged for Mom. Dad was appreciative but it reinforced the fact that Mom was dying. He had never used the actual word and found it very difficult to face. In his mind, he wanted to be the one to control her fate and alter her course but was not allowed that luxury. He denied any services that were not absolutely necessary, and continued to care for her in his own way. His efforts proved to be satisfying yet frustrating due to the anguish of a futile cause.

In May, Mom's shaking spells were more frequent during the night and the drug Atavan was prescribed. She was given one tablet before bed time but later that evening; she became limp and totally unresponsive. Hospice advised taking half a tablet and Dad agonized with alternating dosages then finally refused giving her the medication at all.

In May, Dad finally admits in his notes that:
It looks like the beginning of the end. Hate to think about it.'
He was still reluctant to use the "D" word.

By now, six months had passed and Mom's sore at the base of her spine was still not healing and had become ulcerated. Various treatments had been tried and failed due to her poor health and circulation so a Foley catheter was inserted to help keep the area dry. It was agonizing to watch

Mom waste away when she had been so vibrant and energetic and worse for Dad who had dedicated his life to her comfort and welfare. She had been so physically healthy. They could have traveled and reaped the benefits of retirement in their 'golden years' but instead, the thievery of Alzheimer's disease had reduced Mom to a fragile shell, as delicate as a whisper.

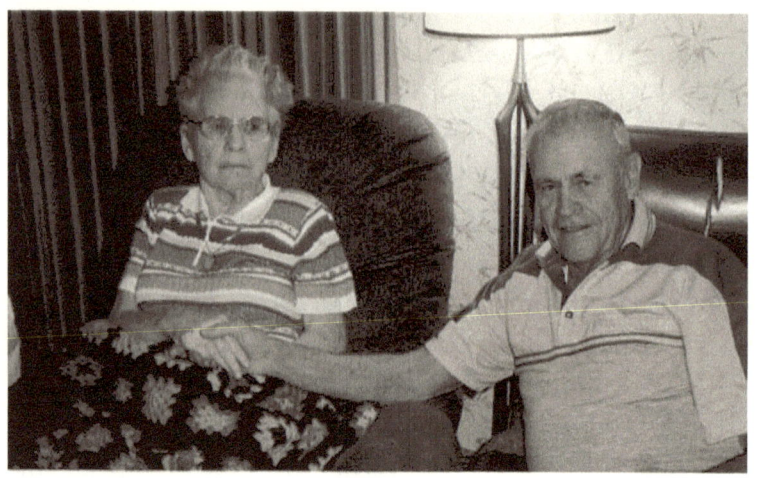

Final anniversary, 59 years together. March14, 2004.

Saturday morning, July 24, 2004, Dad was amazed at how alert Mom seemed. She would not eat, but appeared calm and at peace. He took her for a ride to Mechanic Falls and she held her head high, looked around, smiled and was more awake than she had been in months. Later that morning, I came over and noticed a distinct change as well. Her eyes were so clear and her face was exceptionally smooth. As I sat with her alone, I held her hand and looked straight into her eyes. It was time for me to say good bye. She honestly looked as though she was waiting to hear my words so I said, "I love you so much, Mom. We all do, but you can go now. I promise you, we will take care of Dad. Dad will be OK, Mom. Dad will be OK." I repeated these lines several times and she never broke her gaze. Her head would nod, her eyebrows twitched and she actually smiled! She could not have presented me with a greater gift. I felt like she trusted my confidence and was more likely to rest. I left for home later that day with a mixed feeling of strength and sadness.

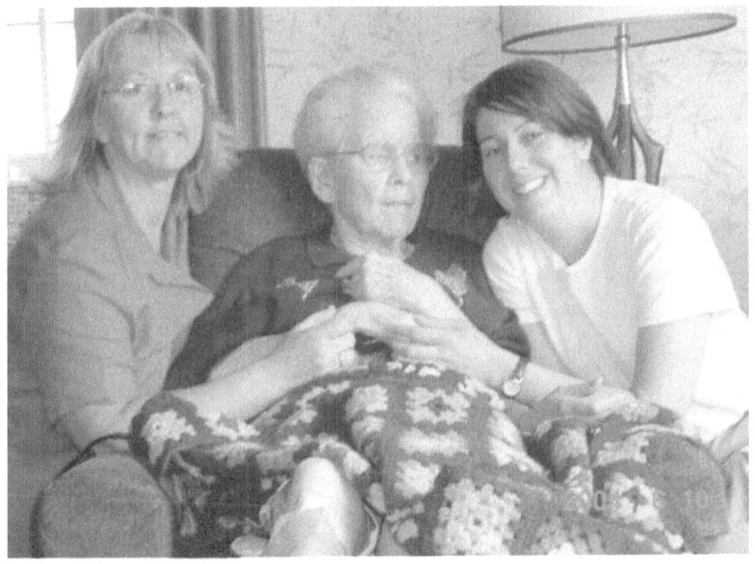

Doris, PCA; Bea and Karyn, hospice nurse. May 2004

The next morning, I received a phone call from the hospice nurse saying Mom had taken a turn for the worst during the night and was nonresponsive. I remember feeling fear, uncertainty, pain, relief and guilt for the entire ride over. Once we arrived, Dad was sitting on the porch with the nurse and my sister. The morning was heavy with doom as we accepted the fact that Mom would never get out of bed again.

All we could provide for her at this time was love, comfort and freedom from pain. She had shriveled down to approximately 70 pounds and needed frequent repositioning to keep her skin from breaking down. Her skin was pasty, her pulse was weak but her respiration was steady. I spent the next few days and nights at the camp feeling fortunate that I could be there for Dad to bathe her in the mornings so that he could avoid looking at her ravaged body. It was a pitiful sight. She was as weak as a baby bird.

Her room was situated directly off of the living area so even when no one was in the room, there was always someone nearby. The next week was like a living wake at home. People would visit Dad, and then pay their respects to Mom who could still hear their words and feel their compassion. Even my dog made frequent visits to her bedside, stretching her neck towards her pillow and then walking away, often settling down near her door way. Dad would often sit on a small stool at her bedside, hold her hand, rub her head and cry. He had no idea how the pain and agony he had suffered over the past 15 years would dull in comparison to the horrific loss he would experience during this final week.

On Monday, July 26th, Mom looked feeble and exhausted. She was dehydrated from being unable to take anything by mouth and Dad finally realized how much control he had lost. "Are we supposed to just wait and watch her die?" he would ask. There was really nothing anyone could do other than reposition her with pillows every two to three hours, rub her back and feet, speak soothingly to let her know we were there and make sure her Foley was draining properly. Her eyes remained open halfway and she was breathing from her mouth, shallow breaths that would cease at short intervals.

As fate would have it, my younger sister Elaine who lived in Texas, had planned a vacation months ago for this particular week in July but her vacation time was abruptly altered for bereavement leave. We wondered whether she would make it here in time at all but as it turned out, she was able to see Mom for the last time. My older sister Anita had also made her peace with Mom in her own private way. She had a special connection because she resembled Mom the most and had been especially close in earlier times.

It was Tuesday night, July 27, when Elaine sat at the head of Mom's bed and cried while thanking her for teaching her how to sew and how to stand up for herself. Her words actually made Mom open her eyes and look up towards the sound of her voice and force a weak smile. She had heard from her youngest and had responded. Her heart was still alive and well.

That night, with Dad's firm resolve to share her bed, he faced her as she once again looked directly at him then weakly moved her hand over his arm. Dad was so distressed that he left the room sobbing and unable to catch his breath. His grief had exposed his vulnerability and he presumably suffered a panic attack. I had just returned home when I received the call from Elaine saying, "I think we're losing Dad!" By the time I arrived back to the camp, the episode was over and he was resting comfortably, but the next morning he admitted his greatest fear at that moment was dying before Mom.

On Wednesday, July 28, the hospice nurse arrived. Mom's color was pale and her pulse was 84. Dad still clung to shreds of hope, knowing in his heart, there was none. No one could assuage his emptiness and despair.

The nurse returned on Thursday, July 29 and remarked there had been little change except for an increased pulse of 102. Her body was working hard to compensate but could not compete with mortality. We all wondered what it was that sustained Mom for so long. Each night I would go to bed praying for the agony to end. I was staying at the lake and would go for a late night swim, look up at the stars and wish Mom could be there too. The stillness of the night seemed so much more appropriate for her now. New days and fresh beginnings had lost their purpose but by Friday morning, Mom lingered on and even managed another feeble smile. Her Foley catheter kept draining 100 to 200cc's of urine each day, defying logic because she had not taken any fluids for weeks and had absolutely no swelling.

Saturday afternoon, July 31, her breathing had become more labored and her pulse was erratic. My sister and I had called Dad in from outside to come in and check on her. Elaine compared her to a tiny fish out of water, gasping for breath. We decided it may be time to administer liquid morphine to keep her comfortable but neither my sister nor I wanted to be the one responsible for possibly giving her a narcotic that could arrest her respirations because she had lost so much weight and we were not sure of the dosage. We spoke with a hospice nurse who encouraged us to give her a small dose and we made a 'pact' between us to each give her two drops of the morphine inside her cheek to be absorbed. It seemed to relax her although her respirations remained labored and shallow. That evening as we sat with Dad on the porch, he mentioned that he had decided to use a Mausoleum rather than a burial site because he did not want to put her body in the ground.

Sunday morning, August 1, a different hospice nurse came to visit. She engaged Dad in casual, pleasant conversation and offered comfort with her casual and caring attitude. Rather than focus on Mom and the hopelessness of her situation, this particular nurse spoke with Dad in the present tense offering genuine compassion and understanding. She quietly asked permission to see Mom and entered the room with utmost respect. She addressed Mom by name and then carefully touched her as if she were made of glass. She took her blood pressure which was 80/40 but was unable to detect an accurate reading for a pulse. Mom was comatose and unable to appreciate the loving care this wonderful young nurse gave her but I believe Mom was being repaid for the same type care she had bestowed upon her many patients during her own nursing career.

The sun rose as on any other day, on Mon August 2. As usual, following Mom's morning care, I repositioned her onto her side, and while doing so, my dog wandered into the room. She had never been allowed on any furniture, but on this particular day, she placed her front paws on the mattress, panting furiously with her ears pulled back flat against her head. I had only seen her react this way during thunderstorms but this morning had dawned cloudless and serene. She could obviously sense a different kind of turbulence.

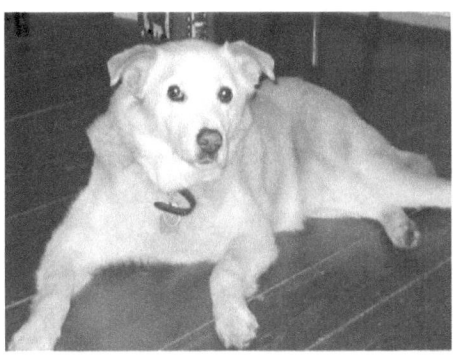

Later that day, I took time to go home and mow my lawn but felt apprehensive about leaving the camp. I decided to go anyway and had visions of how much Mom had enjoyed being outdoors and mowing her lawn in the past. She worked fast and efficiently and as I pushed my own lawn mower, I asked her to please wait until I finished before going anywhere. I assumed she would understand. When I returned to camp, she had not changed. Another hospice nurse had come and this time, she could not obtain her B/P and there was 50cc's of urine in her drainage bag. Her major organs were shutting down and she was fading rapidly. Relatives continued to pass through with condolences and empty words of courage, but essentially, it was up to Mom to give the last call.

At 9 PM, Mom lay on her left side as the cords in the back of her neck appeared exceptionally pronounced. The outline of her profile was sharp with her sunken eyes and jutting cheek bones. Her skin was cold and her slim fingers were cyanotic as we tried in vain, to bundle her for warmth. The mask of death had made her nearly unrecognizable. She began to make moaning sounds with her breathing as forced air rushed over her vocal cords. It had been several months since we had heard Mom's voice and hearing it in this artificial manner was very disturbing. More morphine was given to ease the stressful breathing and the mournful sound stopped. By 10 PM, her beautiful blue eyes glazed over and Mom took her last breath surrounded by her family and Dad at her side as he had been for nearly 60 years. The anticipation of her death did not prepare us for the finality of the moment. I felt that my Mom was aware of my Dad's presence as she let herself go beyond her earthly pain and suffering. Her lifeless body seemed to sink into the bed as her muscles relaxed and her body succumbed to defeat while her spirit joined the stars. Her battle was over. Mom was free and both of Dad's wishes had been granted.

The final entry in Dad's notes was written the next day on August 3, 2004.

Trying hard to live without Bea. I will miss her dearly.

Mom's funeral was on August 6, 2004 at 11AM. As the procession of cars wound its way towards the church, the hearse paused for a moment in front of the house where Mom and Dad had lived. I was so proud of my father's stamina and determination on that day. He humbly claimed that his exceptionally good health and the quality care he gave my Mother would have been impossible without the support of his loving family, the dedicated staff of Androscoggin Home Health and Mom's very special personal care attendant, Doris. He claims, "They were always there if I needed them."

I wrote this memoir of my mother to ease my own personal grief and to bless her memory, but the main reason was to present this tribute in writing to my Dad with the hope that he can obtain a glimpse of how he was perceived by those closest to him and accept the credit for his outstanding perseverance. Dad, I hope you can believe you were the guardian angel on earth that Mom could feel, hear and recognize. She was never alone and what mattered the most was that at the end, someone who loved her sat by her, saying, "I still see you."

Afterward

I will always admire my Dad's generous heart and enduring tenacity for in spite of the discouraging course of my mother's wretched disease, he remains strong enough to honor her with distinction and continues to do so by visiting her grave every day, and embracing her memory by presenting her with a red rose and kissing her beloved name engraved in the stone.

Still Here

Do not try to find, where I have gone,

I'm someone different, far beyond.

And although I may look to be quite the same

I am slowly forgetting your face and your name.

I've lost the ability and the means

To express the horrible way that I feel.

But your words and your touch, I do sense

They bless me with love and confidence.

So please be patient and repeat in kind

Respond as if for the very first time.

And if I pretend that I already knew,

I'm just trying to hide my shame from you.

And there will be times when I'll seem not to care,

But blame my disease for being unfair.

I wish words would come to help you understand

Yet my voice remains silent while my heart is in your hand.

~ Suzanne Johnson

About the Disease

I graduated from nursing school in 1971, at a time when Alzheimer's was even more of a mystery than it is today. Back then, it was often linked with dementia which is primarily caused by a hardening of the arteries, while Alzheimer's has a distinctive feature of a buildup of amyloid plaques on the brain, causing brain functions to shut down over a course of time. I am ashamed to admit that during the 70's, Alzheimer's patients did not receive the care and attention they deserved. It was assumed that old age harbored dementia and Alzheimer's patients were listed as such.

The nursing home I worked at in 1972 had no special unit for Alzheimer's patients. They were often restrained in chairs and rolled out into large solariums to be left there until it was time for someone to feed them a meal. Heavy doses of sedatives were frequently administered to healthier individuals who managed to wander outdoors or become belligerent. Some of the patients were ridiculed by the younger aides who did not know any better. I distinctly remember a retired teacher we had as a patient. Every morning, she was bathed and harnessed into her chair with wheels and parked near the nurses' station. She believed she was still a teacher and would often speak to the staff as if they were her pupils. It was endearing to most, but in retrospect, she was worthy of much more care and respect than she received.

Personally, I am angry and frustrated with this growing disease. It completely dissolved my mother and devastated my father in ways unimaginable. Their "golden years" were tarnished with the pain and restrictions caused by Alzheimer's. We, as a family, were bewildered by the new roles we had to learn while my mother was forced into a frightening world of delusion and stolen from us at a precious time when my own children were growing up.

Hopefully research will find a cure for this menacing disease before the next generation.

To this day, there is still no cure for Alzheimer's Disease, but we have learned that Alzheimer's patients suffer a sense of fear and detachment that is incomprehensible to healthy individuals. It begins with a sense of loss, confusion and disorientation, and then proceeds to episodes of paranoia, often leading to drastic personality changes and death. Imagine being trapped in a glass box with no one but strangers in foreign languages tending to your needs. Or worse, imagine the glass box.

Recently, there have been new medications developed to delay the onset of Alzheimer's. Studies are currently being made on the blood brain barrier which consists of a layer of cells that line the inner walls of the cranial blood vessels. This barrier blocks the passage of toxins, while allowing oxygen, sugar and other nutrients to the brain. If scientists can find a way to penetrate the blood brain block so that medication can pass directly to the affected portion of the brain, we may be able to dissolve the plaques and harness the disease. Amyloid beta proteins are responsible for the formation of plaques on the brain related to Alzheimer's. However, these proteins are unable to cross the barrier unless they attach themselves to a much larger molecule known as RAGE. (Receptor for Advanced Glycation End product) This process also reduces normal blood flow to the brain aggravating brain degeneration. By disabling the RAGE molecule through genetic engineering, it is possible that the damaging amyloid protein will be unable to anchor itself to the brain, thus preventing the dreaded disease.

Resources

The Alzheimer's Association (National Organization)

www.alz.org – Website for the Alzheimer's Association

The Alzheimer's Association, the world leader in Alzheimer research and support, is the first and largest voluntary health organization dedicated to finding prevention methods, treatments and an eventual cure for Alzheimer's. Phone: 1.800.272.3900.

Local Chapters of the Alzheimer's Association

http://www.alz.org/findchapter.asp

For Caregivers

http://www.alz.org/Care/overview.asp

This site provides the caregiver with information to care for the person with dementia and to care for themselves.

Caregiver kit (request from your local library)

A video series featuring caregivers and their families talking about their experiences caring for their loved ones with Alzheimer's disease. Titles are: Meeting Daily Challenges, Communicating, Safety First, Managing Difficult Behavior, and Caring for the Caregiver.

5 videocassettes (93 min); learning guide, caregiver packet

Order no. ED 248Z, items may be purchased separately.

800.272.3900.

www.ingramcontent.com/pod-product-compliance
Lightning Source LLC
Chambersburg PA
CBHW020402290526
45785CB00005B/2406